Issouf IRA

Post-traumatic peritonitis

Issouf IRA

Post-traumatic peritonitis

ScienciaScripts

Imprint

Any brand names and product names mentioned in this book are subject to trademark, brand or patent protection and are trademarks or registered trademarks of their respective holders. The use of brand names, product names, common names, trade names, product descriptions etc. even without a particular marking in this work is in no way to be construed to mean that such names may be regarded as unrestricted in respect of trademark and brand protection legislation and could thus be used by anyone.

Cover image: www.ingimage.com

This book is a translation from the original published under ISBN 978-620-6-72029-4.

Publisher:
Sciencia Scripts
is a trademark of
Dodo Books Indian Ocean Ltd. and OmniScriptum S.R.L publishing group

120 High Road, East Finchley, London, N2 9ED, United Kingdom
Str. Armeneasca 28/1, office 1, Chisinau MD-2012, Republic of Moldova, Europe
Printed at: see last page
ISBN: 978-620-8-02403-1

DEDICACES & THANKS

SIGNING SESSIONS

To the Eternal God

Glorified be you who keeps us breathing the breath of life in good health. You began this work that you continue to perfect for your glory. Eternal One, my flesh and my heart may be consumed, but you will always be the rock of my heart and my portion.

To my Dad Ira Itiédouin and my Mum Lallou Mamina in Dâ *Thank you for all the sacrifice you have made to get me here. This work is dedicated to you, the fruit of your determination. You have always provided me with a good education and your advice has raised me to this level. You have always encouraged me and steered me in the right direction. Thank you for your confidence in me during my studies. I love you all very much.*

To my Papa Koné Aboubakar Sidiki and all the family in Côte d'Ivoire

You've set a good example for me to follow. Here are the results, and you should be honoured, because this work is yours. You gave absolutely your best so that I could reach this level. I love you very much and thank you again for your constant love.

To my uncle Ira Honoré and his wife

Thank you, my parents in the faith of Christ. You have always taught me common sense and love of neighbour. I dedicate this work to you.

To my aunts, brothers and sisters, cousins

Your support was crucial to the success of my work. You have always in a good family atmosphere. I dedicate this work to you.

To my darling Davou Awa

You have been a profound source of inspiration for me. You have always had faith in me and supported me constantly. This work, the fruit of our love, is dedicated to you. Thank you for your patience.

ACKNOWLEDGEMENTS

To General Lougué and his wife Pr Lougué, to Dr Loué and his wife
Thank you for guiding me along this path and making it easier for me to get there. You have had faith in me and given me your support throughout my journey.
At the Assemblies of God church in Songnaaba

You were the host family I needed to make this project a success. work. Thank you for all your support.

To my elders: Dr Coulibaly Batan Roland, Dr Tamini Kansi Bienvenu, Dr Ilboudo Mahamadi, Dr Kouglo R. Boris
Thank you, dear elders, for your advice and guidance. You gave me a lot of support throughout the process and in the preparation of this work.
My classmates: Mme Ouédraogo / Tiemtoré Sampawendé Dielle Firmie, Bado Léticia Pélagie, Illo Sonia Carine Philette, Bancé Aïcha, Bontouré P M Josepha, Bonkoungou Fleur, Ilboudo Daniel, Ilboudo Fabrice, Guissou Michael, Tindano Daniel, Lougué Kouamé, Sourou Bédimè Robert,
Thank you for all your support during the development of this work.

To Bassinga Adama (In memoriam):

You were a model comrade for me. You gave me a lot of support. Thank you for everything.

TO OUR MASTERS AND JUDGES

To our teacher and Chairman of the jury: Professor Maurice Zida
You are

- o *Full Professor of Visceral Surgery at the University's UFR/SDS Joseph Ki-Zerbo ;*

- o *Surgeon visceral at Centre Hospital University Hospital Yalgado Ouédraogo University Hospital;*

- o *Head of the General and Digestive Surgery Department at the Yalgado Ouédraogo University Hospital;*

- o *Colonel Major of the National Armed Forces of Burkina Faso ;*

- o *Knight of the National Order ;*

- o *Technical adviser in charge of security issues for the Ministry of Health.*

Dear Master,It is a great pleasure and an honour for us to have you sit on this jury, despite your busy schedule. We were lucky enough to benefit from your theoretical and practical teaching during our training. Your extensive scientific knowledge, your availability and your great human qualities have won our admiration. The time spent at your side has enabled us to discover in you a man of research who cares deeply about the training of students. Your modesty, your rigour in your work and your availability make you a teacher appreciated by all. Dear Master, allow us, on this day, to express our gratitude to you. May the Lord God Almighty continue to multiply his wonders in you,may he watch over you and your family. Amen to that!

TO OUR MASTER THESIS DIRECTOR: PROFESSOR EDGAR OUANGRE

You are

o *Full Professor of General Surgery at the University's UFR/SDS Joseph Ki-Zerbo ;*

o *Surgeon General at Centre Hospital Universitaire Yalgado Ouédraogo ;*

o *Head of the Visceral Emergency Unit at the Yalgado Ouédraogo University Hospital;*

o *President of the Burkinabe Society of Surgery (SOBUCHIR) ;*

o *Knight of the National Order of Merit of Burkina Faso;*

o *Vice-Chairman of the Centre's Medical Committee*

Yalgado OUEDRAOGO University Hospital ;

o *Director General of the Ecole Nationale de Santé Publique.*

Dear Master,

It is an immense pleasure and an honour for you to have entrusted us with this work and to have generously agreed to guide us, in spite of your multiple occupations. We were fortunate to benefit from your theoretical and practical teaching during our training period in the general and digestive surgery department of the CHU-YO. Your extensive scientific knowledge, your availability and your great human qualities have won our admiration. The time we spent with you enabled us to discover that you were a man of research who was very concerned about the training of students. Your simplicity, your love of teaching and your rigour in practical training make you a great hope for current and future generations of doctors. Dear Master, we are at a loss for words to express our gratitude and profound appreciation. May God shower you and your family with his abundant graces. We pray Amen!

A OUR MASTER MEMBER OF THE JURY : DOCTOR DOAMBA RODRIGUE

Namekinsba

You are

o *Assistant in General Surgery at the UFR/SDS of the University Joseph Ki Zerbo ;*

o *Former intern at the Ouagadougou Hospitals;*

o *Former Foreign Resident of the Paris Hospitals;*

o *General and hepato-bilio-pancreatic surgeon at the Tengandogo University Hospital.*

Dear Master,

We would like to express our gratitude to you for having spontaneously agreed to take part in this thesis jury despite your very busy schedule. Your immense scientific knowledge, your rigour in your work and your human qualities command our respect, as we have had the opportunity to benefit from your teaching during our studies. Please accept, dear Master, the expression of our deepest respect and our sincere thanks.

May the Lord Almighty shower you and your family with his rich blessings. your family. Amen to that!

WARNING

By deliberation, the UFR/SDS has decided that the opinions expressed in the essays to be submitted must be considered as the authors' own and that it does not intend to give them any approval or disapproval.

TABLE OF CONTENTS

INTRODUCTION AND STATEMENT OF THE PROBLEM

Peritonitis is the acute inflammation or infection of the thin membrane covering the intra-abdominal organs. It is generally secondary to perforation of a hollow digestive organ or to the spread of an intra-abdominal septic focus. It may be generalised or localised[5,11].

Acute generalised peritonitis accounts for a large proportion of abdominal emergencies. According to Clément et al, it is a global health problem, with a mortality rate of up to 20%[15]. In 2020, Tochie et al. reported a worldwide prevalence of 0.93% and a mortality rate ranging from 8.4% to 34%, depending on the country and the aetiology [51].

According to the Hamburg classification, peritonitis can be primary, secondary or tertiary. Secondary peritonitis is the most common, accounting for 98% of peritonitis and 7% of abdominal pain syndromes. It may occur following abdominal trauma, contusion or injury to the abdomen, per endoscopic perforation or the presence of an intra-abdominal foreign body. It is a surgical emergency, and the prognosis remains serious, depending on the patient's general condition and the absence of early and appropriate resuscitation [10,13,16,46].

Despite appropriate resuscitation, abdominal trauma is still a public health problem, with the occurrence of peritonitis increasing the mortality rate to 12% or even 18% [24]. In Europe, post-traumatic peritonitis occurs mainly as a result of road traffic accidents, which are the most frequent cause of abdominal trauma[52]. The incidence is thought to be higher in Africa, where there is growing insecurity. In Morocco, Elasbahani Y. in 2020 found a prevalence of 12.5% in a series of 109 cases [22]. In abdominal contusions, Raherinantenaina F. et al found a prevalence of peritonitis of 84.3% and 47.07% in wounds. in a series of 175 cases in Madagascar [43].

In Chad, Choua O. found a prevalence of 46%, which represented 15.15% of visceral surgical emergencies in 2017. And depending on the series, mortality rates vary between 25% and 63% in developing countries[14].

In Mali, Sogba et al found a prevalence of 2.39% in a series of 256 patients [48]. Diakité L. found 2.4% in a population of 42 patients [18]. Magagie A. et al found 8.52% of post-traumatic peritonitis in a study of 622 patients operated on for digestive surgical emergencies, with a morbidity of 38.10%, dominated by post-traumatic peritonitis in 2016 in Niger [32]. Burkina Faso, which shares the same health and security realities with these two countries, has the same proportions of peritonitis.In rural Burkina Faso, we found 1.8% of post-traumatic peritonitis in 2013 according to Ouangré E. et al[36]. But in urban areas, Kaboré E. reported a prevalence of 14% at the Centre Hospitalier Universitaire Tengandogo (CHU-T) in 2018 [27]. At the Centre Hospitalier Universitaire Yalgado Ouédraogo (CHU-YO), Daboué in 2016 had a prevalence of 6.6% and Ilboudo F. found 3.46% in 2019 [16,25]. In 2020, Ouédraogo I. found 3% [38]. Attiou T. O. in 2020 at CHU-T, 23.9% in abdominal gunshot wounds with a 5.2% mortality rate, dominated by peritonitis [3]. In Burkina Faso, post-traumatic peritonitis is reported to be on the increase as a result of growing insecurity and violent abdominal trauma. The lack of rapid and appropriate treatment worsens the prognosis. Also, since the Daboué studies in 2016, we have very little data on the subject in our context despite the apparent increase in the number of cases. This prompted our study.

PART I

GENERAL

1. DEFINITION

1.1. Definition

The peritoneum is an intra-abdomino-pelvic membrane covering the viscera. It is a smooth, transparent serosa made up of two layers. A parietal sheet which lines the intra-abdominopelvic wall and a visceral sheet which covers all or part of the surface of the intra-abdominopelvic viscera [12,17,21].

1.2. Reminder anatomy

The peritoneum is the serosa that lines the inside of the abdominal and pelvic cavity, Figure 1 [47]. It is made up of mesothelial tissue. This tissue consists of a flattened cell layer with a polygonal outline. The cell layer rests on a basement membrane in direct contact with a connective stroma. This connective stroma contains vascular, nervous and lymphatic elements. The two layers of the peritoneum are organised in a particular way within the abdominal cavity [30].

1.2.1 The parietal sheet

The parietal layer, also known as the parietal peritoneum, lines the inside of the abdominal cavity, Figure 4 [44]. It distinguishes four parts of the abdominal cavity.

o A diaphragmatic part located at the top, richly vascularised

and innervated. It causes hiccups when irritated.

o An anterior part that forms the pre-peritoneal space with the abdominal wall.

o A posterior part which forms the retroperitoneum with organs behind the peritoneum. These organs are partially covered. These are the large vessels, the abdominal aorta and the inferior vena cava.

The urinary tract, with the kidneys and ureters, and the adrenal glands are in this zone. The duodenum and pancreas are also found here.

o And a pelvic part in the pelvis, which forms the cul de sac of Douglas in front of the rectum.

The parietal layer is vascularised by the vessels of the abdominal wall and is also innervated by the nerves of the abdominal wall [7,12,13,21,23].

11

1.2.2 The visceral layer

Also known as visceral peritoneum, it is in direct contact with the organs it covers, the intraperitoneal organs, figure 3 [44]. It covers the stomach, liver, spleen, small intestine and colon. It covers the viscera by forming folds. These folds have various names.
o A ligament, when they connect an organ to the abdominal wall, such as the falciform ligament of the liver.
o A meso, when they form the attachment of an organ to the wall, such as the meso of the transverse colon.
o An omentum or epiploon when they connect two organs, the greater and lesser omentum.
The meso of the transverse colon defines two zones.

o The sub-mesocolic zone, where the greater omentum covers the lower abdomen. the small intestine like an apron.

o The supramesocolic area, where the small omentum is found.

The visceral peritoneum, like the parietal peritoneum, is vascularised by the vessels of the viscera it covers. It is innervated by the nerves of the organs it covers [7,12,13,21,23].

1.2.3 The peritoneal cavity

The parietal and visceral layers of the peritoneum delimit a space called the peritoneal cavity, located in the abdominal and pelvic cavity, figure 2 [44]. The peritoneal cavity is completely closed in men. In women, it communicates with the tubal canal via the abdominal ostium of the uterine tube. It is a space containing a thin film of fluid of approximately 50 cubic centimetres, facilitating the mobility of the two sheets and of organs intrapéritonéaux [7,12,13,21,23].

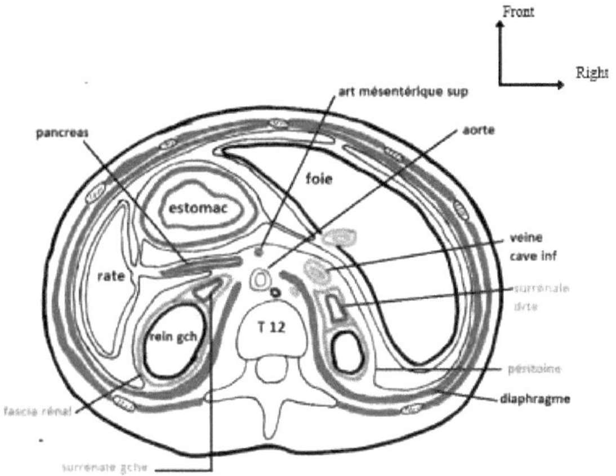

Figure 1: Cross-section of the abdomen through T12

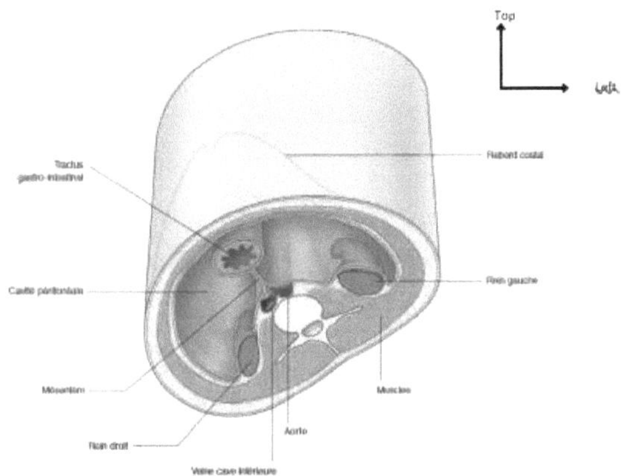

Figure 2: Lower view of abdominal contents

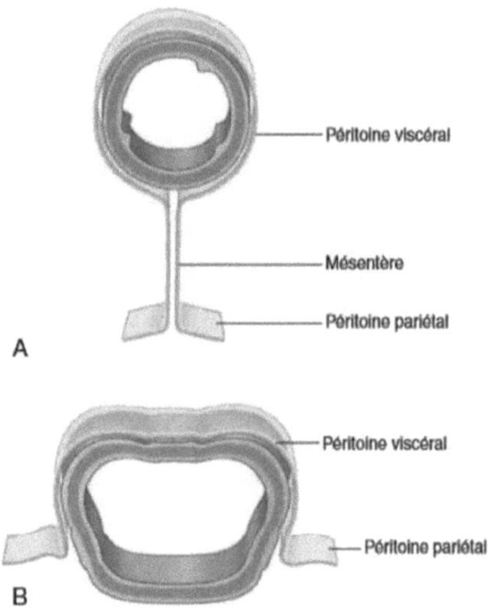

Figure 3 : A = Intraperitoneal. B = Retroperitoneal.

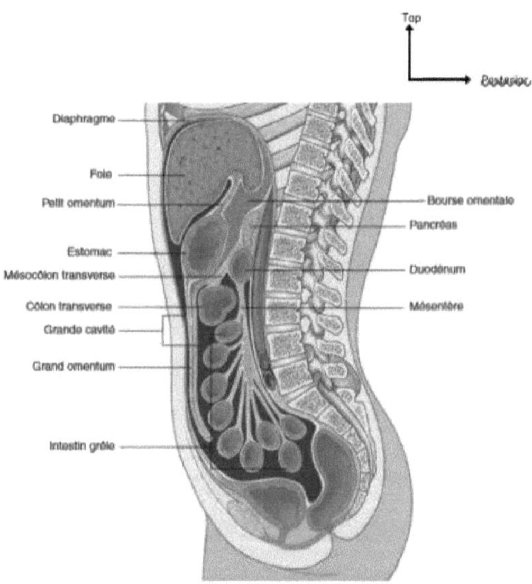

Figure 4: Side view of abdominal contents

1.3. Etiopathogenesis of peritonitis

1.3.1 Function of the peritoneum

The peritoneum has four essential functions:

o It secretes fluid from the interstitial fluid. It stores around 50 cm^3 of this secretion in the peritoneal cavity to facilitate the sliding of the two sheets.
o The peritoneum is a semi-permeable membrane. It therefore performs a resorption function. It has a surface area of around 1700cm^2 and can absorb 450ml/h of liquid and small molecules.
o It has a defence function. This function is made possible by the presence of defence cells in the peritoneum.
o It also has a plastic function, with the ability to renew and repair itself. It is the integrity of its basement membrane that enables this function [5].

1.3.2 Mechanism of inflammation of the peritoneum Inflammation of the peritoneum may be bacterial from the outset as a result of the spread of an infectious site, or chemical following perforation o f   a hollow intra-abdominal organ.

In abdominal trauma, the initial attack is chemical, followed by a secondary bacterial attack. The consequences of this aggression are both local and general [23,35].
o Locoregionally, there is an intense inflammatory reaction. This reaction leads to intraperitoneal exudation, with accumulation of fluid in the peritoneal cavity. It also leads to paralytic ileus, resulting in the creation of a third sector.
o On a general level, there will be a reduction in circulating blood flow.

This will lead to a reduction in blood perfusion in certain organs, resulting in anoxia. Anoxia therefore leads to hyperventilation and an increase in heart rate. This whole phenomenon explains all the clinical and psychological manifestations of the disease. of peritonitis [2,17].

1.3.3 Traumatic causes of inflammation of the peritoneum Abdominal trauma results from an acute transfer of energy that exceeds the body's physiological capacity for resistance. This transfer of energy can cause open trauma to the abdomen or closed trauma to the abdomen. Closed trauma to the abdomen, or contusion of the abdomen, occurs when there is no break in the continuity of the abdominal wall [7]. They occur in particular in :

o Road traffic accidents account for the majority of abdominal injuries [4,45]. The victims include pedestrians, cyclists, motorcyclists and occupants of motor vehicles.

o Falls from height can be intentional, as in the case of autolysis, or unintentional.

o Physical assaults, particularly in brawls.

o Cattle kicking and hoof beating

Open trauma to the abdomen results in a break in the continuity of the abdominal wall. They cause either a penetrating abdominal wound, which is a wound of the abdomen with effraction of the peritoneum, or a perforating wound of the abdomen when the viscera are affected [7]. They are mainly encountered in :

o Abdominal stab wounds are the main cause of open trauma to the abdomen. It is involved in physical assaults and autolysis.

o Abdominal injuries caused by firearms are on the increase as a result of insecurity. They cause multiple intra-abdominal injuries, depending on the type of projectile. An exit wound is always sought.

o Traffic accidents with high impact energy.

2. STUDY CLINICAL

2.1. Type of description : Generalized acute peritonitis, sthenic form

2.1.1. Initial assessment

On admission, the patient is questioned about the nature of the trauma, the nature of the vulnating agent, and the time of onset of the trauma, with abdominal pain in the foreground.The initial emergency assessment consists of looking for signs of haemodynamic instability. Blood pressure (BP), heart rate (HR), respiratory rate (RR) and conjunctival colouration are assessed. During this initial assessment, preoperative resuscitation is started and blood is taken for additional emergency tests. At this stage, vomiting of food or biliousness may be noted, as well as a disorder of the intestinal transit due to paralytic ileus [35].

2.1.2. General examination

The patient's general condition deteriorates rapidly, unless early and appropriate resuscitation is given, as a result of multiple organ failure. There is an infectious syndrome, with hyperthermia at 39°C or even 40°C, or sometimes hypothermia, tachycardia and polypnoea [35].

2.1.3. Physical examination

Examination of the abdomen is the essential part of the diagnosis. It is carried out on an unclothed patient lying supine on a hard surface. The arms are at the sides of the body, the thighs are slightly abducted and the legs are semi-flexed.

o At the inspection

The abdomen is immobile and not breathing. The rectus abdominis muscles are contracted and protrude under the skin. We look for points of impact, bruising, excoriations and abdominal wounds. In abdominal wounds, we look for an entry hole and an exit hole, especially in the case of firearm trauma.

o On palpation

It is performed gently, with the hands warmed and placed flat on the skin. the abdomen.

She finds the abdominal contracture, which is an involuntary rigidity of the abdominal wall. It is tonic, permanent, invincible, painful and produces a

wooden stomach. It can be replaced by a generalised abdominal defence, which is triggered by deep palpation and which can be overcome with gentle and progressive palpation. Palpation of the umbilical region reveals the umbilical cry, which is a sharp pain triggered by sudden decompression of the umbilicus.
o Percussion

The flanks may be dull if there is a peritoneal effusion. Pre-hepatic dullness disappears in the event of gas effusion in the the peritoneal cavity.

o On auscultation

Intestinal sounds are reduced or absent, indicating a cessation of intestinal peristalsis.
o On rectal examination

There is the Douglas cry, which is a sharp pain triggered by rectal examination [1,12,17].

2.1.4. Additional examinations

Post-traumatic acute generalised peritonitis (AGP) is a surgical emergency and no further investigation should delay its management.
o Biology

•The haemogram is used to look for anaemia, especially in the presence of haemodynamic instability. Hyperleukocytosis or leukopenia may also be present in the presence of an infectious syndrome.
•We are trying to determine the rhesus blood group for a possible blood transfusion.
Biochemistry is used to assess renal function, blood sugar levels and the existence of a hydrolytic disorder on the blood ionogram [17].

o Imaging

•An unprepared abdominal X-ray (APX) revealed pneumoperitoneum, which was consistent with perforation of a hollow organ. It is characterised by a gas crescent between the hepato diaphragm on the right and under the phrenic on the left.
Sometimes, the gaseous crescent overlies a liquid effusion.

X-rays may also reveal diffuse greying [2].
•Abdominal ultrasound can detect intra-abdominal fluid effusion and check the integrity of solid intra-abdominal organs [9].

• Abdomino-pelvic computed tomography replaces the X-ray of the PSA. It can be used to detect signs that cannot be seen on the X-ray. It can be used to correct the diagnosis when the clinical examination is doubtful, by demonstrating pneumoperitoneum or an intra-abdominal fluid effusion. It may also reveal an intra-abdominal foreign body [12,17].

2.1.5. Evolution without treatment

This development is not conceivable in a hospital environment. It leads to septic complications.

o Locally, there are intra-abdominal abscesses.

o Distant liver, kidney and brain abscesses can occur.

All of these complications progress to death through multivisceral failure. **[17]**.

2.2. Clinical forms

2.2.1. Symptomatic form

o Sthenic peritonitis

The sthenic form of peritonitis, as described here, is dominated by abdominal pain.
On clinical examination, the main symptom is contracture. abdominal muscles with a wooden belly.

o Asthenic peritonitis

In the asthenic forms, the symptomatology is frugal.

Abdominal pain is persistent, but abdominal contracture is replaced by generalised abdominal defence. The Douglas cry is not obvious on rectal examination. These forms occur in patients with a profound deterioration in general condition. It occurs in patients who have consulted a specialist late after abdominal trauma, as well as in post-traumatic PAG in patients with an underlying defect [12].

2.2.2. Topographical shapes

In post-traumatic GAP, the topography varies according to the area of the digestive tract affected in the peritoneal cavity. Perforation occurs as a result of direct impact or the fall of pressure sores [29].

o The stomach: Because of its position between the cardia and the pylorus, it can burst in contusions of the abdomen from front to back, pressing against a rigid plane formed by the spine and ribs. In the region of the epigastrium, it is also exposed in abdominal blunt trauma.

o The small intestine: It occupies a large part of the peritoneal cavity. This exposes it to trauma, which can cause peritonitis. The duodenum is limited between the pylorus and the duodeno-jejunal angle. Compression of the duodenum in abdominal contusions can cause it to burst. The jejunum and ileum are the most frequently involved in abdominal wounds.

o The colon: This is a highly septic area. Perforation rapidly causes infection of the peritoneum. This means that surgical treatment generally involves digestive bypass.

o Trauma to the hypogastric region includes intra- or sub-peritoneal bladder rupture. These lesions are diagnosed by intravenous urography.

2.2.3. Associated shapes

Lesions of the intraperitoneal hollow viscera may be isolated or associated with to other lesions.

o Intra-abdominal solid viscera: the liver and spleen are generally found in abdominal trauma in association with the injury. intra-abdominal hollow viscera, table I [6].

o In polytrauma, we find several other associated injuries: limb fractures, pelvic fractures, spinal injuries and brain injuries.

The patient's vital prognosis is compromised when there is a combination of injuries, particularly in polytrauma patients.

Table I: Intraoperative discovery
Isolated lesions organ

Damaged organs	Percentage (%)
Small intestine (jejunum and/or ileum)	24,3
Stomach	2,7
Rectum	5,4
Epiploon	2,7
Diaphragm	2,7
Small + colon	8,1
Small intestine + liver	5,4
Small intestine + vascular wound	5,4
Epiploon + stomach	5,4
Small intestine + colon + bladder	2,7
Small intestine + Rectum Associated lesions	2,7
Epiploon + small intestine	2,7
Diaphragm + spleen + stomach	2,7
Diaphragm + liver	2,7
Spleen + colon	2,7
Small intestine + spleen	2,7
No lesions	16,2

3. DIAGNOSIS OF POST-TRAUMATIC PERITONITIS

3.1. Diagnosis positive

A positive diagnosis should not delay resuscitation. Clinical examination is sufficient to make the diagnosis of post-traumatic peritonitis: peritoneal syndrome occurring after trauma. In frustratingly symptomatic forms, radiological assessment is essential for diagnosis.

3.2. Diagnosis differential

The differential diagnosis of post-traumatic peritonitis is post-traumatic haemoperitoneum. It occurs in cases of injury to solid intra-abdominal organs, particularly the liver and spleen. It can be ruled out in the absence of a frank peritoneal syndrome and on abdominal CT scan.

4. Treatment

4.1. Goal

The aim of treatment in post-traumatic GAP can be divided into three parts:
- Early correction of the disorders and general consequences of peritonitis
- Treatment of inflammation of the peritoneum

- Removal of the cause of the peritonitis [12].

4.2. Resources and methods

3.2.1. Medical treatment

It is always indicated and is carried out during hospitalisation, with the patient

is put on an empty stomach.

o Resuscitation

It must be adapted and undertaken rapidly as soon as the patient is admitted.

• It consists of inserting two good-calibre peripheral or central venous lines, a nasogastric tube and a urinary catheter.

• In the event of haemodynamic instability, with abnormal central venous pressure, heart rate and blood pressure, vascular filling with macromolecules is initiated. In the event of severe anaemia due to haemorrhage, an iso rhesus group blood transfusion is carried out.

• Oxygen therapy will be started if peripheral oxygen saturation is unsatisfactory.

• The correction of electrolytic disorders must not be delayed.

Rehydration should be undertaken to prevent possible renal failure, which could occur in the context of hypovolaemia.

Resuscitation continues before, during and after the operation.

o Antibiotic therapy

It begins as soon as the diagnosis is made and is administered parenterally as a synergistic combination.

It must be broad-spectrum from the outset, directed against Gram-negative bacilli.

and anaerobic bacteria [40].

There are several possible schemes:

• A combination of Amoxicillin + Clavulanic Acid and Aminoside
• A combination of third-generation cephalosporins and imidazoles
• A combination of Imidazoles and Aminoside

It is then adapted to the results of bacteriological tests and continues postoperatively.

o Other resources

• Analgesics are administered during resuscitation. In general, level II analgesics from the WHO classification of analgesics.

• Serotherapy and anti-tetanus vaccination are undertaken in all patients with open trauma who are not up-to-date with their anti-tetanus vaccination.

• Stress digestive ulcers and digestive haemorrhage are prevented by administering a Proton Pump Inhibitor (PPI) and enteral feeding as soon as possible.

• Thromboembolic disease must be prevented by administering fractionated heparins at iso-coagulant doses [12,42].

3.2.2. Surgical treatment

Although it is the principle treatment for peritonitis, it is undertaken in a patient who has received medical resuscitation.The approach is a median laparotomy under general anaesthetic with orotracheal intubation.All liquids will be sampled for bacteriological analysis. present at the opening of the abdominal cavity. The peritoneal cavity and all the intra-abdominopelvic organs are fully explored. Perforations are treated according to their diameter and the segments of the digestive tract affected.An ostomy will be performed if there is a serious infection.If false membranes form in the abdominal cavity, they are removed. Abundant peritoneal cleansing is carried out with warm isotonic saline (approximately 10 litres). Finally, the abdominal wall is closed with a drain placed in the down position. This drain allows the serohaematic fluid that oozes into the peritoneal cavity after the operation to drain outwards [12].

3.2.3. Post-operative care

Post-operatively, the aim is to continue resuscitation and monitor vital functions. Pain management continues Antibiotic therapy i s continued, adapted to the results of the swabs. bacteriological. The surgical wound must be monitored and treated

4.3. Indication

Post-traumatic GAP is a clear indication for emergency laparotomy, with early medical resuscitation tailored to the patient. Serotherapy and tetanus vaccination are indicated in all patients with open trauma and is not up to date with their tetanus vaccination. At laparotomy, the organ affected is usually repaired, depending on the lesion. There is no anastomosis in a septic environment at ileal level, in which case a stoma is performed [12,35,41].

4.4. Duration of treatment

Resuscitation is continued until vital signs have returned to normal with a clinical and biological monitoring. Analgesic treatment continues for at least seventy-two hours after the operation. The duration of antibiotic treatment is either fixed at between five and seven days, or variable depending on the clinical and biological evolution.

4.5. Evolution and surveillance

3.5.1. Surveillance elements

Post-operative monitoring covers :

o General signs: haemodynamic constants, pain, ventilatory function, diuresis and body temperature are monitored.

o Local signs: we monitor the condition of the dressing, the resumption of bowel movements, the state of the stomach, etc. drain and stoma.

o Biology: the haemogram is used to check that the number of polymorphonuclear cells has returned to normal and that haemoglobin levels have increased.

A blood ionogram is used to check that the disorders have returned to normal. hydroelectrolytics.

3.5.2. Post-operative complications

The complications, linked to the severity of the trauma and the delay in treatment, are :

o Parietal suppuration

o Haemorrhage and haematoma

o Post-operative peritonitis

o Post-operative occlusions

o Post-operative ventrations or eviscerations

o Persistence or recurrence of an infectious phenomenon

o Stoma malfunction

o Wall abscesses.

3.5.3. Prognosis

Post-traumatic peritonitis has a serious prognosis.

o It depends on the severity of the trauma and the associated injuries: polytrauma.

o The prognosis is guarded in colonic cases and in immunocompromised patients.

o It also depends on how early appropriate and effective treatment is provided.the patient's age [31].

PART II

27

1. OBJECTIVES

1.1 General objective

To study post-traumatic peritonitis in the general and digestive surgery department of the Centre Hospitalier Universitaire Yalgado Ouédraogo (CHU-YO) from 1er April 2019 to 31 March 2022 in order to improve management

1.2 Specific objectives

1. To determine the frequency of post-traumatic peritonitis in the general and digestive surgery department of the Centre Hospitalier Universitaire Yalgado Ouédraogo from 1er April 2019 to 31 March 2022.
2. To determine the circumstances of occurrenceZQ4 of post-traumatic peritonitis in the general and digestive surgery department of the Centre Hospitalier Universitaire Yalgado Ouédraogo from 1er April 2019 to 31 March 2022.
3. To determine the sociodemographic aspects of patients admitted for post-traumatic peritonitis in the general and digestive surgery department of the Yalgado Ouédraogo University Hospital Centre from 1er April 2019 to 31 March 2022.
4. To describe the diagnostic aspects of post-traumatic peritonitis in the general and digestive surgery department of the Centre Hospitalier Universitaire Yalgado Ouédraogo from 1er April 2019 to 31 March 2022.
5. To evaluate the results of the management of post-traumatic peritonitis in the general and digestive surgery department of the Yalgado Ouédraogo University Hospital Centre from 1er April 2019 to 31 March 2022.

2. METHODOLOGY

2.1. Framework of the study

2.1.1. Burkina Faso

Located in West Africa, in the loop of the Niger, Burkina Faso is a landlocked country with no maritime outlet. It borders Ghana, Togo and Benin to the south, Niger to the east, Mali to the north and Côte d'Ivoire to the south-west. Its climate is intertropical, of the Sudano-Sahelian type, with alternating seasons of unequal length. A dry season lasting eight to nine months from October to May and a rainy season lasting three to four months from May to September. It is therefore subject to climatic hazards, particularly droughts and floods, as well as the harmattan [53]. According to the United Nations Development Programme (UNDP) report for 2021, it is one of the developing countries, ranking 184^{em} out of 195 countries in the world [54]. And according to the Institut National de la Statistique et de la Démographie (INSD), in 2021, 41.4% of its population will be living below the poverty line.Administratively, it is divided into 13 regions, 45 provinces, 370 départements, 351 communes (49 urban and 302 rural) and 8,438 villages. The regions are headed by governors, the provinces by high commissioners and the communes by mayors.According to the INSD report, the population of Burkina Faso in 2022 is estimated at 20,505,155 people, distributed as 75.1 inhabitants/km^2 . Men account for 48.3% and women for 51.7%. It is predominantly rural, with 73.9% of the population living in rural areas. The fertility rate is 5.4 children per woman. Its birth rate is 39.4‰ [38]. Since 1993, Burkina Faso has adopted the district system as the basis of its health system. It is administratively subdivided into three levels

o A central level represented by the cabinet of the Ministry of Health, the general secretariat and the technical departments

o An intermediate level corresponding to the regional health directorates

o And a peripheral level represented by the health districts.

In operational terms, the health system takes the form of a pyramid with three levels.

o The 1er level is the health district, which is subdivided into two levels

• The 1er level is the health and social promotion centre (CSPS). In 2020, Burkina Faso had 201

• The 2^{em} level is the medical centre with a surgical unit (CMA) or district hospital. There will be 46 CMAs in 2020

o The second level is the regional hospital centre (CHR), which serves as a reference for the CMAs. There were 09 of these in 2020, and they provide what is known as secondary care.

o The 3^{em} level is the university hospital centre (CHU), which serves as a reference for the RHCs and provides so-called tertiary care. There will be 06 of these by 2020, including 04 in Ouagadougou.

There are also private health establishments, mainly located in the cities of Ouagadougou and Bobo Dioulasso. In 2020, there were 165 private health establishments.

The Centre Hospitalier Universitaire Yalgado Ouédraogo is one of the 04 CHU located in Burkina Faso. in Ouagadougou.

2.1.2. Yalado Ouédraogo University Hospital (CHU - YO)

Built in 1961, the Centre Hospitalier Universitaire Yalgado Ouédraogo is one of the leading hospitals in Burkina Faso. It receives patients from Ouagadougou, the surrounding provinces and even further afield. In order to meet the health needs of the population, its areas of activity have gradually expanded and diversified. It is now subdivided into 10 departments:

o The Department of Medicine and Medical Specialities

o The Department of Surgery and Surgical Specialities

o The laboratory department

o The radiology and nuclear medicine department

o The anaesthesia and intensive care department

o The odontostomatology department

o The obstetrics and gynaecology department

o The paediatrics department

o The hospital pharmacy department

o The Public Health Department

It provides a training environment for doctors in specialisation, medical and pharmacy students, senior laboratory technicians and paramedical staff. The General and Digestive Surgery Department is one of the departments in the Department of Surgery and Surgical Specialities.

2.1.3. General and digestive surgery department

In the Department of Surgery and Surgical Specialties, the General and Digestive Surgery Department is where our study took place. It is located to the east of the Yalgado Ouédraogo University Hospital. It accepts patients aged 15 and over and comprises three units:
o Visceral emergencies, which include

- A reception room with a capacity of six beds

- An observation room with 14 beds

- Two first category observation rooms

- An operating theatre with two operating theatres

- A dressing room

- A depot for medicines and emergency kits

o The operating theatre unit consists of three operating theatres shared with the urology department, plus a sterilisation room.
o An inpatient unit with a capacity of 48 beds. It accommodates post-operative patients as well as those awaiting elective surgery. This unit also houses staff consultation and meeting rooms.
Its medical staff consists of :

o A full professor of general surgery

o A full professor of visceral surgery

o A senior lecturer in surgical oncology

o Six hospital surgeons

Its paramedical staff consists of :

o 19 health attachés in anaesthesia and intensive care

o 10 qualified nurses and 7 registered nurses

o 12 stretcher-bearers

o From seven boys and girls in the hall

o A secretary

It is organised as follows:

o Therapeutic activities such as :

•Outpatient consultations, Monday to Thursday

•A general visit every Friday, led by the Head of Department

•Daily visits from Monday to Friday by a surgeon

•Scheduled surgery on Mondays, Tuesdays and Thursdays

•A duty and on-call programme

o Training and research activities as part of initial and continuing training, as well as supervising doctors enrolled for the Diplôme d'Etudes Spécialisées (DES) in general and digestive surgery.

o Educational activities such as :

•Discussion and teaching sessions from Monday to Friday

•Weekly presentations by doctors enrolled in the DES, as well as by interns and externs from the $3^{\text{ème}}$ year of medicine to the $6^{\text{ème}}$ year.

As part of its training activities, the department brings together doctors enrolled in postgraduate courses in general and digestive surgery, medical students from the Health Science Training and Research Unit (UFR/SDS) at Joseph Ki Zerbo University, and students from the private Catholic University of Saint Thomas Aquinas (USTA). Finally, the department provides practical training for trainees from the National School of Public Health (ENSP).

2.2. Materials and method

2.2.1. Type of study

This was a descriptive cross-sectional study with retrospective data collection.

2.2.2. Study population and study period

Our study focused on the records of patients received for abdominal trauma and hospitalised in the general and digestive surgery department of the CHU-YO during the period from 1er April 2019 to 31 March 2022.

o **Inclusion criteria**

Our study included all patients consulted in the general and digestive surgery department of the Centre Hospitalier Universitaire Yalgado Ouédraogo (CHU-YO) in whom the diagnosis of post-traumatic peritonitis was made on the basis of clinical and paraclinical arguments and intraoperative findings during the study period and who had a complete file.

o **Non-inclusion criteria**

Patients operated on for post-traumatic peritonitis whose records were incomplete or could not be found were not included in our study.

2.2.3. Data collection and analysis

A pre-test was carried out to evaluate our data collection and analysis tools.

This evaluation was carried out on six patients between 23 and 25 November 2022.

Data collection took place in the general surgery department

and digestive systems at CHU-YO, from 28 November 2022 to 23 December 2022

Socio-demographic, clinical, para-clinical, therapeutic and evolutionary data were recorded on a survey form for patients included in the study from :

o The register of visceral emergencies and general and digestive surgery

o Surgical report book

o Records of patients operated on for post-traumatic peritonitis

o The patient discharge register for the general and digestive surgery department.

The data were entered and analysed on a microcomputer using EPI INFO software (French version 7.2.2.6), Microsoft Excel 2016 and Microsoft Word 2016.

2.2.4. Study variables

o The socio-demographic variables are: age in years, gender (male or female), place of residence (rural or urban), occupation

o The clinical variables are: reason for consultation, admission time, pathological history (medical and surgical), functional signs, general signs and physical signs of the disease.

o Paraclinical variables include: CBC (leukocytes, haemoglobin level, platelets), PSA (gas crescent, hydroaerobic level, diffuse greyness).

o The therapeutic variables are: the intervention time in hours, the treatment administered (preoperative resuscitation, antibiotics, analgesics and postoperative), surgical technique, intraoperative diagnosis (aetiology of the peritonitis) and the surgical procedure.

o The evolutionary variables are: the outcome of the treatment (simple continuation or postoperative complication), postoperative complications (parietal suppuration, evisceration, postoperative peritonitis, digestive fistula, postoperative occlusion), length of hospital stay in days and mode of discharge (cured, death).

2.2.5. Ethical and administrative considerations

In accordance with Article 158 of the harmonised codes of ethics and practice, medical records remain the private property of the hospital service. Thus, the confidential nature of patient data and anonymity are respected in our study. First and foremost, we requested authorisation to carry out the study from the head of the CHU-YO and the general and digestive surgery department.

2.2.6. Definitions of terms

Admission delay: this is the time elapsed between the trauma and admission to the hospital. the visceral emergency department of the CHU-YO.

Time to surgery: this is the time elapsed between admission to the visceral emergency department and the start of surgery.
Polytrauma: a patient with two or more serious traumatic injuries, at least one of which is life-threatening in the short term.
Shock: acute circulatory failure that permanently alters the oxygenation and metabolism of tissues and organs.

3. RESULTS

3.1 socio-demographic data

3.1.1 Frequency

From 1er April 2019 to 31 March 2022 we recorded 56 cases of post-traumatic peritonitis. During the same period, we recorded 164 cases of abdominal trauma, 698 cases of acute generalised peritonitis and 3,429 cases of abdominal emergencies.

Post-traumatic peritonitis accounted for 34.14% of abdominal trauma, 8.02% of acute generalised peritonitis and 1.6% of surgical abdominal emergencies.

In Figure 5 we have represented the frequency in the form of a diagram

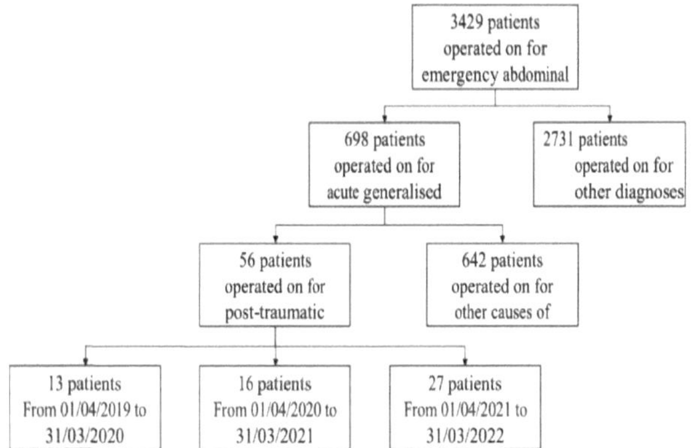

Figure 5: Flow chart

3.1.1 Annual repairs

The average annual number of post-traumatic peritonitis cases was 18. The breakdown by year is shown in Figure 6.

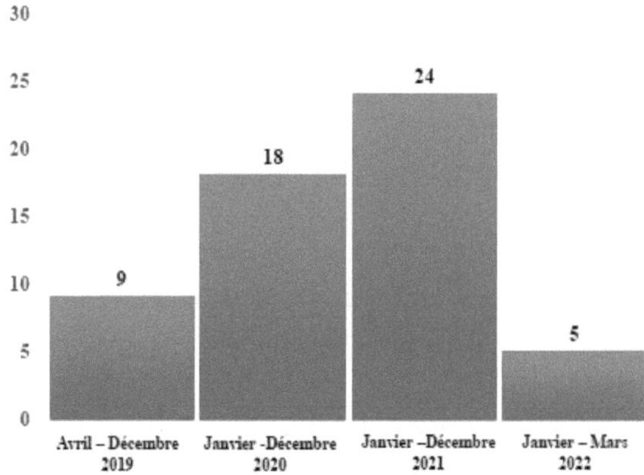

Figure 6: Annual distribution of patients. N=56

3.1.2 Monthly repairs

The monthly breakdown gives an average of four cases per month. Figure 7 shows the monthly breakdown of patients.

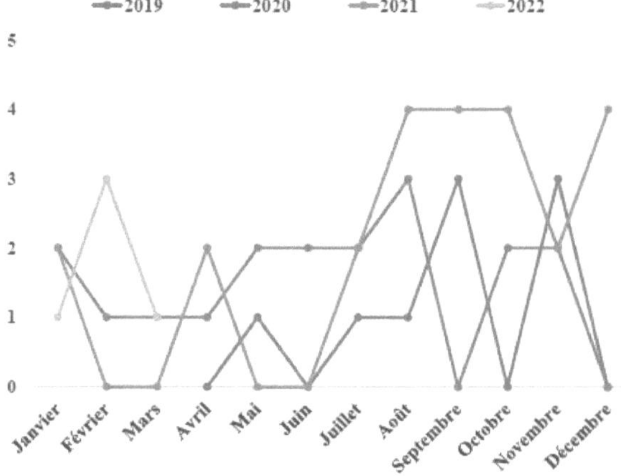

Figure 7: Monthly distribution of patients. N=56

3.1.3 Age

Of the 56 patients, the mean age was 30.39 years, with extremes of 15 years. and 57 years of age. The breakdown by age group is shown in Figure 7.

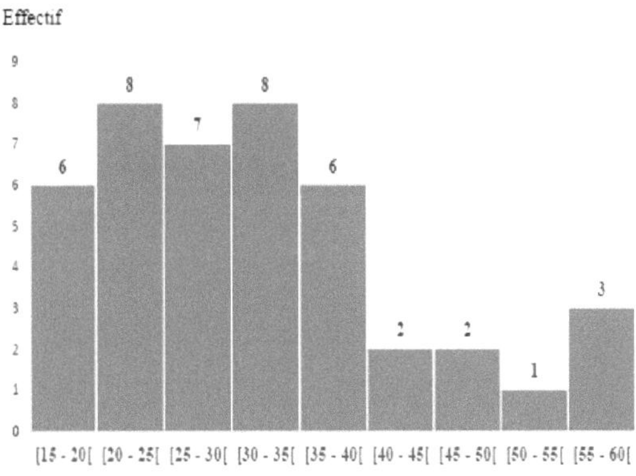

Figure 8: Breakdown of patients by age group. N=56

3.1.4 Socio-professional activity

Occupation was specified for all 56 patients. The breakdown is given in Table II

Table II: Socio-professional distribution of patients. **N=56**

Socio-professional activity	Workforce	Percentage (%)
Informal sector	24	42,85
Farmer / Breeder	13	23,21
Pupil / Student	11	19,64
Employee	6	10,71
Housewife	2	3,57
Total	56	100

3.1.5 Sex

Sex was recorded for all our patients. We recorded 53 men (94.64%) and three women (5.36%). The sex ratio was 17.66.

3.1.6 The residence

In our study, 37 patients (66.07%) lived in urban areas and 19 (33.9%) in rural areas.

3.1.7 Admission procedure

Table III shows the distribution of patients by mode of admission, and Table IV shows the distribution of patients by referral structure.

Table III: Breakdown of patients by mode of admission. N=56

Admission procedure	Workforce	Percentage (%)
Reference	42	75
Direct	11	19,64
Transfer	3	5,36
TOTAL	56	100

Table IV: Breakdown of patients by referral structure. n=42

Reference structure	Workforce	Percentage (%)
CMA	22	52,38
CHR	12	28,57
CHU	2	4,76
FS Private	6	14,29

CHR Regional Hospital Centre CHU University Hospital Centre
CMA Centre Médical avec Antenne chirurgicale FS Privée:Formation Sanitaire Privée

3.2 Data

3.2.1 The consultation period

The distribution of patients according to the time taken for consultation is summarised in Table V. The average delay was seven point seven hours, with extremes of one hour and one month.

Table V: Distribution of patients according to consultation delay. N=56

Consultation period	Workforce	Percentage (%)
[0 - 6h[	46	82,14
[6am - 12pm[	4	7,14
[12h - 1 month]	6	10,71
TOTAL	56	100

3.2.2 Antecedents

In our study, we found one patient (01.7%) with a history of hernia repair surgery. Alcohol consumption was noted in 12 patients (21.42%) and smoking in 10 patients (17.85%).

3.2.3 The reason for consultation

Table VI shows the repair of patients according to the reason for consultation. Open trauma accounted for 50% and closed trauma for 50%.

Table VI: Breakdown of patients by reason for consultation. N=56

Reason for consultation	Workforce	Frequency (%)
Abdominal pain	56	100
Contusion	28	50
Abdominal wound	22	39,29
Evisceration	6	10,71

3.2.4 Circumstances of occurrence

Table VII shows the distribution of patients according to the circumstances in which the trauma occurred.

Table VII: Distribution of patients according to circumstances of onset. N=56

Circumstance of occurrence	Number	Percentage (%)
Stabbing	16	28,57
Assault with a firearm	7	12,5
Car and motorbike accidents the abdomen	3	5,35
Hunting accident	1	1,78
Landslide	1	1,78
Motorbike accident - obstacle	15	26,78
Motorbike accident - motorbike	7	12,5
Sports accident the abdomen	3	5,35
Bludgeon	2	3,57
Falls from height	1	1,78
Total	56	100

3.2.5 The vulnating agent

The distribution of patients according to the vulnating agent in the occurrence of the trauma is shown in Table VIII.

Table VIII: Distribution of patients according to vulnating agent. N=56

Agent vulnérant		Effectif	Pourcentage (%)
Contusion de l'abdomen	Objet contondant	23	40,07
	Ballon de football	3	5,35
	Répression par coup de matraque	2	3,57
Plaie de l'abdomen	Objet tranchant	17	30,35
	Projectile	8	14,28
	Eboulement	1	1,78
	Chute de hauteur	1	1,78
Total		56	100

3.2.6 General examination

The distribution of patients according to the results of the general examination is summarised in Table IX

Table IX: Distribution of patients according to general examination. N=56

Examen		Effectif	Pourcentage (%)
Etat général	Stade II	31	55,35
	Stade III	25	44,64
Etat de conscience	Normal	56	100
Conjonctives	Normo colorées	54	96,42
	Pâle anictérique	2	3,57
Température	Hyperthermie	12	37,5
	Hypothermie	1	1,78
Tension artérielle	Hypertension	4	7,14
	Hypotension	3	5,35
Fréquence cardiaque	Tachycardie	19	33,92
Fréquence respiratoire	Tachypnée	14	25
Pouls	Petit et Filant	2	3,57
Etat hémodynamique	Etat de choc	2	3,57

3.2.7 Physical examination

o **Inspection**

The inspection revealed an anomaly in 44 patients, as shown in Table X.

Table X: Distribution of patients according to inspection results. n=44

Inspection	Workforce	Percentage (%)
Abdominal wound	22	39,28
Abdominal distension	21	37,5
Post-traumatic evisceration	06	10,71

o **Palpation**

The results of palpation are shown in Table XI

.**Table XI:** Distribution of patients according to palpation findings. N=56

Palpation	Workforce	Percentage (%)
Cry of the umbilicus	25	44,64
Generalised abdominal defence	24	42,85
Abdominal contracture	10	17,85

o **Percussion**

We found tympany on percussion in eight patients (14.28%) and sloping flank dullness in seven patients (12.5%).

o **Auscultation**

Auscultation revealed abdominal silence in seven patients (12.5%).

o **Rectal touch**

A rectal examination revealed a Douglas cry in 11 patients (19.64%).

3.2.8 Associated lesions

Abdominal trauma was associated with injuries in 13 patients (23.21%). The breakdown is given in Table XII

Table XII: Distribution of patients according to associated lesions. n=14

Associated lesion	Workforce
Limb fracture	5
Excoriation / bruising	7
Pelvic fracture	1
Ruptured spleen	1

3.3 Paraclinical data

3.3.1 Haematological check-up

Haemogram results showed hyperleukocytosis in 17 patients (30.35%) and leukopenia in three patients (5.35%). Anemia was found in seven patients (12.5%).

3.3.2 Biochemical check-up

Biochemistry revealed hyperglycaemia in six patients (10.71%) and hypoglycaemia in two patients (3.57%). Serum creatinine was elevated in eight patients (14.28%) and urea in five (08.92%).

3.3.3 Blood ionograms

On the blood ionogram, we found an ion disorder in one patient hyponatremia.

3.3.4 Imaging results

An unprepared abdominal X-ray was performed in two patients and found a gaseous crescent in both, i.e. 100%. Abdominal ultrasound was performed in 19 patients and found haemoperitoneum in 16 (84.21%). Abdominal CT scans were performed in four patients. It revealed a gaseous crescent in two patients (50%) and a liquid effusion in two patients (50%).

3.4 Data

3.4.1 Resuscitation and medical treatment

In our study, all patients received preoperative care. The distribution of patients according to preoperative resuscitation is given in Table XIII.

Table XIII: Distribution of patients according to preoperative care received.
N=56

Care administered	Workforce	Frequency (%)
Rehydration	56	100
Nasogastric tube	56	100
Urinary catheter	56	100
Venous route	56	100
Nefopam	55	98,21
Paracetamol	54	96,42
Metronidazole	29	51,78
Ceftriaxone	29	51,78
Tetanus serotherapy	8	14,28
Amoxicillin clavulanic acid	2	03,57
Tramadol	2	03,57
Blood transfusion	1	01,78
Vascular filling	2	03,57

3.4.2 Time to surgery

The delay in surgical management for our patients is summarised in Table XIV. The average delay was 21.83 hours, ranging from 30 minutes to seven days.

Table XIV: Distribution of patients according to time to surgery. N=56

Delays in surgical management	Workforce	Percentage (%)
[0 - 6h[	5	8,82
[6h - 24h[	25	44,64
[24h - 48h[	22	39,29
[48h - 7jours[	4	7,14
TOTAL	56	100

3.4.3 Anaesthesia method

All our patients underwent surgery under general anaesthetic with orotracheal intubation.

3.4.4 The approach

The approach consisted of a median incision above and below the umbilicus in all our patients.

3.4.5 Exploring

The distribution of patients according to the nature of the aspiration fluid is summarised in Table XV. In all cases, a sample of the fluid was taken and sent for cytobacteriological study.

Table XV: Distribution of patients according to cavity condition and the nature of the aspiration fluid. n=47

Type of suction fluid	Workforce	Percentage (%)
Serohaematic fluid	22	39,28
Bile fluid	10	17,85
Fecal fluid	9	16,07
Serous liquid	3	5,35
Purulent fluid	3	5,35
Total	47	83,92

The distribution of patients according to the organs injured is summarised in Table XVI.

Table XVI: Distribution of patients according to organ damage. N=56

Damaged organ	Workforce	Frequency (%)
Jejunum	33	58,92
Iléon	13	23,21
Colon	10	17,85
Stomach	3	05,35
Bladder	2	03,57

3.4.6 Surgical procedures performed

Table XVII shows the distribution of patients according to the procedures performed.

Table XVII: Breakdown by surgical procedure. N=56

Action taken	Workforce	Frequency (%)
Peritoneal cleansing	54	96,42
Aspiration of abdominal fluid	47	83,92
Small suture excision	22	39,28
Small bowel anastomosis resection	21	37,5
Removal of false membranes	14	25
Ileostomy	7	12,5
Colon anastomosis resection	3	5,35
Gastrorraphy	3	5,35
Epiplasty	2	3,57
Excision colon suture	2	3,57
Associated gesture		
Fracture trimming	4	7,14
Splenectomy	1	1,78

3.4.7 Post-operative care

Post-operative medical care is summarised in Table XVIII.

Table XVIII: Distribution according to postoperative care. N=56

Care administered	Workforce	Frequency (%)
Rehydration	56	100
Paracetamol	56	100
Nefopam	55	98,21
Ceftriaxone	52	92,85
Metronidazole	48	85,71
Anticoagulant	35	62,50
PPI	19	33,92
Gentamycin	9	16,07
Amoxicillin clavulanic acid	4	7,14
Tramadol	1	1,78

PPI Proton Pump Inhibitor

3.5 Data from

3.5.1 The evolutionary aspect

In our study, 50 patients, i.e. 89.29%, had a simple post-operative course. Six patients (10.71%) had complicated postoperative recovery. Three patients (5.35%) were re-operated following complications. Table XIX shows the various complications.

Table XIX: Distribution of patients according to postoperative complications.
N=06

Complications		Effectif
Complications spécifiques	Péritonite post opératoire	2
	Eviscération post opératoire	1
	Suppuration pariétale	1
Complications générales	Sepsis	1
	Escarres	1

3.5.2 Mortality

We found two cases of death, representing 3.57%. The first case of death occurred after a general complication such as sepsis in a context of delayed consultation. The second case of death occurred after a specific complication in the form of postoperative peritonitis. The patient was 57 years old and had multiple lesions.

3.5.3 Output mode

The breakdown by mode of exit is summarised in Table XX

Table XX: Breakdown of patients by mode of discharge. N=56

Exit mode	Workforce	Percentage (%)
Healed	53	94,64
Transferred	1	1,79
Deceased	2	3,57
TOTAL	56	100

3.5.4 Length of hospital stay

Table XXI summarises the distribution of patients by length of hospitalisation. The average was 11.83 days, with extremes of four days and 32 days.

Table XXI: Breakdown of patients by duration of treatment hospitalization.
N=56

Length of hospital stay	Workforce	Percentage (%)
<5 days	4	7,14
[5 days - 10 days[	37	66,07
[10 days - 20 days]	11	19,64
>20 days	4	7,14
TOTAL	56	100

3.5.5 Monitoring

In the follow-up, 54 patients (96.42%) were seen again two weeks after discharge and showed a favourable outcome.

4. COMMENT AND DISCUSSION

4.1 Limits and constraints

Our study encountered a number of difficulties, including the following:

✓ The poor lighting in the archive room made it difficult to search through patient files;
✓ Lack of information on certain patients in the admissions register;
✓ Information missing from certain files ;

✓ The absence of results of paraclinical tests in certain patients;

✓ The operative report register was insufficiently completed for some patients;
✓ Lack of data on the post-operative follow-up of patients;

✓ The scarcity of studies on post-traumatic GAP was one of the major difficulties in our study.
Despite these limitations and constraints, which have marred our work, we have achieved results that we will discuss below.

4.2 Socio-demographic aspects

4.2.1 Frequencies

In the literature, there are very few reports of post-traumatic PAG. They represented 08.02% of PAG in our study, i.e. 56 out of 698 patients treated for PAG. They accounted for 34.14% of abdominal trauma in visceral emergencies at the CHU-YO. In the same department, our results are better than those of Daboué [16] and Ilboudo [25] who found 6.6% and 3.46% of PAG respectively. These differences could be explained by the country's deteriorating security context during our study period. Elsewhere, Kaboré [27] found a higher prevalence than ours, 14% at CHU- T In Niger, our rate is close to that of Magagie [32], who found a rate of 8.52%. In Mali, Sogba et al [48] found a prevalence of 2.39%, which is well below our result. The annual distribution of peritonitis shows an increasing prevalence. From 2019 to 2021, the figures are 16.07%, 32.14% and 42.85% respectively. This can be explained by the security situation, which is worsening year on year. Added to this is ignorance of and non-compliance with the highway code, as well as the dilapidated and narrow nature of some roads. The monthly breakdown shows peaks in August, September, October and November. This can be explained by the rainy season, which leads to a deterioration in the road network, thus favouring the occurrence of traffic accidents.

4.2.2 Age and gender

The mean age of our 56 patients was 30 years, with extremes of 15 and 57 years. Our results are similar to those of Daboué [16], who found an average age of 30.07 years, with a maximum age of 75 years. Our results are lower than those of Ilboudo [25] in Burkina Faso and Diakité [18] in Mali, who respectively have an average age of 38 and 40.1 years. The most representative age groups were [15-20[, [20-25[, [25-30[and [30-35[, with 16.07%, 19.64%, 17.85% and 17.85% respectively. These results are similar to those of Daboué [16] and Ilboudo [25]. This could be explained by the structure of the Burkina population. The population under 40 years of age represents 83.1% of the general population. As young people are the most solicited in all areas of daily life, they are the most exposed to the occurrence of post-traumatic PAG. The sex ratio was 17.66 in our study. This is much higher than that of Daboué [16] and Ilboudo [25], who found 6.67 and 5.5 respectively, and also that of Kambiré [28], which was 13 for abdominal trauma. This large difference could be explained by the greater involvement of men in acts of insecurity such as assaults and brawls.

4.2.3 Socio-professional activity

The informal sector, as reported in the literature, was predominantly represented with 40.07%. Traders dominated this sector. Daboué [16] also found this sector in the lead with a higher rate than ours of 43.68%. But Ilboudo [25], with a lower rate than ours, 31%, also found this sector predominant. On the other hand, in Chad, Choua O [14] finds this sector in third position. This could be explained by the high mobility of traders and their lack of knowledge of the highway code, which exposes them to traffic accidents and their major involvement in brawls. They were followed by farmers (25%) and pupils and students (19.64%) in our study.

4.2.4 Source

We found that 66.07% of patients came from urban areas. This result is similar to that of Daboué [16] who found 63.37%. This could be explained by the population density in urban areas and the development of lifestyles. The assault rate is increasingly high in urban areas [24]. In contrast, Ilboudo [25] found a higher rate of patients from rural areas (51.99%). This can be explained by the fact that insecurity became widespread in urban areas during the period of our study.

4.2.5 Admission procedure

Referral was the most frequent mode of admission in our study, accounting for 75% of patients. This rate is higher than that of Choua O [14] in Chad, who found that 30% of patients were referred. In our context, this large difference can be explained by the pyramid structure of the healthcare system. The population consults at the lower level or in the nearest health centre before being referred to the higher level [37].

4.3 Clinical

4.3.1 The consultation period

The majority of our patients (82.14%) consulted a health facility after their abdominal trauma within six hours. Our results are superior to those of Diarra L [20] in Mali. In the case of traumatic perforation of the digestive tract, he found that 53.3% of patients consulted a health facility within six hours of their abdominal trauma. Our results are also better than those of Sambo [45] in Benin, who found 71% of patients consulted within 24 hours of abdominal trauma. This could be explained by the good organisation of the health system in Burkina Faso, which provides care that is easily accessible to the majority of the population [37]. The severity of abdominal trauma is also a main factor that leads patients to consult a health centre immediately after their trauma.

4.3.2 History

We found alcohol consumption in 21.42% of our patients. This result is lower than that of Daboué [16], who found a rate of 31.68% in his study in 2016. Increased awareness of the harmful effects of alcohol consumption could explain this difference. On the other hand, Ouédraogo [39] in 2020 had a rate of

10.45%, lower than our result. The increase in the standard of living of the general population could explain this difference, with an increasing proliferation of drinking establishments.

4.3.3 Reason for consultation

In 50% of our patients, the reason for consultation was abdominal contusion with abdominal pain. This rate is lower than that of Sylla D [49] in Mali who found 57.14% of abdominal contusion with abdominal pain in post-traumatic digestive perforations. Similarly, Mouzou [34] in Togo found a higher rate of 64.54%. Sambo [45] in Benin found a rate well above ours at 75.5% of cases.
Abdominal trauma by blunt trauma predominated in their studies. In our series, the rate of sharp-force injuries was similar to that of blunt-force abdominal injuries, which would explain these differences.

4.3.4 Circumstances of occurrence

In the circumstances of onset, road traffic accidents are the most common, as in most cases in the literature, with a rate of 44.64%. Sambo [45] in Benin found a lower rate than ours, 31.63%. Also in Mali, Sylla D [49] found a rate of 38.1% in road traffic accidents, which predominates in the occurrence of traumatic digestive perforations. The young age of users of high-speed vehicles, together with the density of road traffic and lack of civic-mindedness, would explain the high incidence of road traffic accidents.After road accidents, we have assaults, which represent 41.07% in our study. While Choua O [14] in Chad found that brawls and assaults were predominant in traumatic perforations of the hollow viscera (69.1%) and road traffic accidents (5%). These rates can be explained by the rise in insecurity due to terrorism and incivism.

4.3.5 Vulnerable agent and nature of the trauma

In 40.07% of cases, the trauma was caused by a blunt instrument. This rate is lower than that of Daboué [16], which found a rate of 76.34% of cases in 2016. This large difference can be explained by the rise in insecurity in recent years, with the increasing involvement of sharp objects in the occurrence of abdominal trauma, as well as projectiles.In our study, 30.35% of peritonitis was caused by sharp objects and 14.28% by projectiles. In Daboué, these rates were 13.98% and 9.68% respectively. In Mali, Diarra L [20] found a rate of 50%, which is higher than our results. Also in Chad, Choua O [14] found that 64.1% of patients suffered abdominal trauma caused by sharp instruments. In our context, road traffic accidents, a source of blunt abdominal trauma, are still frequent despite an increase in the prevalence of sharp abdominal trauma. We found that a firearm projectile was involved in 14.28% of cases. This rate is higher than that of Choua O [14] who found 8.5%. In his population, we note a predominance of bladed weapons, which he explains by the carrying of knives, which is a cultural attribute. However, our results are similar to those of Diarra L [20] and Diamoutene [19] in Mali, who found 16.60% and 15.60% of cases respectively. The security crisis that has been raging in Mali since 2012 and in Burkina during our study period could explain this high rate with the involvement of firearms in abdominal trauma [50].

4.3.6 General signs

In our series, stage II of the WHO performance status classification was predominant in 55.35% of patients and stage III in 44.64%. Conversely, Daboué [16] found a predominance of stage III (67.33%) and stage II (27.72%). This can be explained by the increase in the number of health centres throughout the country since 2016. This would facilitate immediate consultation in a health centre for rapid treatment to prevent a deterioration in the general condition of patients.We found a normal state of consciousness in all our patients, i.e. 100%. On the other hand, Daboué [16] in his series found a normal state of consciousness in 60.4%. The installation of speed bumps on traffic lanes, the wearing of helmets on two-wheeled vehicles and awareness campaigns on compliance with traffic regulations help to reduce the violence of traffic accidents. As a result, patients arrive at the health centres in a good state of mind.In terms of haemodynamics, 3.5% of patients presented with an unstable haemodynamic state. Elasbahani [22] in Morocco found 5.50% of patients with an unstable haemodynamic state in abdominal trauma. This higher rate than ours could be explained by early management in our context where 82.14% consulted immediately after their abdominal trauma.

4.3.7 Physical signs

On physical examination, palpation revealed a cry from the umbilicus in 44.64% of cases, generalised abdominal tenderness in 42.85% of cases and contracture in 17.85% of cases. These rates are higher in paediatrics, as shown by Maiga M B [33] in Mali, who found that 92.3% of her patients presented with a cry from the umbilicus and 71.8% with abdominal contracture. This would indicate that children are more sensitive to pain. The violence of trauma in adults also leads to immediate treatment before the infection spreads. Douglas cry on rectal examination was found in 19.64% of patients. Daboué [16] had a much higher rate than us, with 69.31%.This difference can be explained by the fact that the patients in our series consultedearly in the majority of cases. Only 25% of our patients had other lesions associated with their abdominal trauma. In contrast, Daboué [16] found other injuries associated with abdominal trauma in 61.38% of patients.

4.4 Paraclinical aspects

4.4.1 Biology

In 30.35% of cases, we found hyperleukocytosis in our study. In closed trauma, Ilboudo F [25] found a slightly higher rate of 33%. This could be explained by the delay in consultation in closed abdominal trauma. Elasbahani [22] in Morocco found a higher rate with 45.87% of cases. Patients admitted for observation in abdominal trauma may present with hyperleukocytosis, thus explaining this high rate.We found anaemia in 12.5% of cases. This rate is lower than that of Elasbahani [22] and Daboué [16] who found 16.50% and 35.64% respectively. The violence of the trauma in their series could explain these high anaemia rates.

4.4.2 Imaging

An unprepared abdominal radiograph was taken in two patients. in our series. Pneumoperitoneum was found in 100% of cases. Daboué [16] had a lower rate of 36.63%.Ultrasonography, carried out in 19 patients, found a liquid effusion in the peritoneum in 84.21% of cases. Daboué [16] found 23.53% cases of peritoneal effusion. On abdominal computed tomography, performed in four patients, we found a liquid effusion in the peritoneum in 50% and pneumoperitoneum in 50%. Elasbahani [22] found 15.27% pneumoperitoneum in his study.Our low proportion of patients in whom imaging examinations were could explain the wide variations in our results.

4.5 Therapeutic aspects

4.5.1 Resuscitation and drug treatment

All patients in our series received preoperative resuscitation. Our results corroborate those of Ouédraogo I [39] who found 100% preoperative resuscitation. On the other hand, 14.28% of patients received anti-tetanus serum, whereas Ouédraogo [39] reported 50.74%. This can be explained by the predominance of contusions in our series.

4.5.2 Surgical treatment

o **Time to surgery**

In our series, only 8.82% of patients benefited from treatment. surgery before the sixth hour. According to Sylla D [49] in Mali, up to 73.81% of patients received surgical management within the first six hours. This delay in treatment in our context is justified by the low number of university hospitals that treat surgical abdominal emergencies.

o **Surgical exploration**

In this study, intraperitoneal fluid was serohematic in 39.28% of cases. This rate is higher than that of Daboué [16], which was 13.86%. In paediatrics, Maiga M B [33] also found a low rate of 7.7% in Mali. The fluid was purulent in 5.35% of cases in our study. In Daboué [16], the rate was higher, at 30.69%, and in Maiga M B[33] with a rate of 51.2%. These differences can be explained by the fact that the majority of our patients consulted immediately after their trauma, within the first six hours. The small intestine is the most affected portion at 82.13%, particularly the jejunum at 58.92%. In Mali, Sylla D [49] also found a high prevalence of small intestine involvement at 61.90%, but with a higher ileal involvement at 33.33%. With regard to the hollow viscera, Kambiré [28] also found a predominance of the small intestine in his series with 71.42%. This could be explained by the anatomical organisation of the small intestine, which is easily accessible in assaults, as well as in traffic accidents.

o **Surgical procedures**

In our series, 83.92% of patients had fluid in the peritoneal cavity. All these patients benefited from aspiration of the intraperitoneal fluid. The small intestine was the organ that benefited most from repair. This included 39.29% suture excision and 37.5% anastomosis resection. Sambo [45] in Benin also found that in abdominal trauma, surgery on the small intestine predominated over surgery on the hollow viscera. Similarly, Ouédraogo [39] found a prevalence of surgery on the small intestine of 55.55%. This can be explained by the fact that the small intestine is the hollow viscera most affected by abdominal trauma.

4.6 Evolutionary aspects

4.6.1 Post-operation

We recorded 10.71% complications in our series, with 33.33% of these complications involving postoperative peritonitis. Sambo [45] in abdominal trauma found a lower rate than ours with 8.16% of complications. Choua O [14] had a rate slightly higher than ours, at 11.10%. These high rates can be explained by the delay in consultation and above all the violence of the trauma.

4.6.2 Mortality

We noted a mortality rate of 3.57%. This rate was low in Daboué [16] in 2016 who found 1.98% mortality. Our cases of death occurred in the context of delayed consultation or post-traumatic peritonitis in an elderly patient.

4.6.3 Output mode

In our series, 94.64% of patients were cured and 1.75% were transferred. Our results are similar to those of Daboué [16] who found a cure rate of 96.04%. This can be explained by early and appropriate management.

CONCLUSION

Post-traumatic PAG is relatively common. Road traffic accidents account for the majority of cases of post-traumatic peritonitis. These are followed by assaults, the proportions of which increase in a context of insecurity. Young males are the population most affected. Imaging is rarely used for diagnosis, which is essentially clinical. The part of the digestive tract most affected is the small intestine, mainly represented by the jejunal portion. Delayed referral and the severity of the trauma worsen the prognosis. As a result, mortality remains high.

SUGGESTIONS

Following our study, we came up with suggestions for reducing the frequency and mortality of acute generalised post-traumatic peritonitis. These suggestions are addressed to different structures:

o **To the Minister for Security**

- Strengthen security measures in urban areas, by stepping up remote surveillance using public surveillance cameras.
- Ensuring that legislation on carrying firearms is enforced, and applying penalties to offenders.

o **To the Minister for Transport**

- Develop a fluid road network with a system for reducing speed.
- Encourage public transport by developing public transport facilities.
- Ensure compliance with the rules of conduct in traffic, by raising awareness and enforcing the law against offenders.

o **To the Minister of Health and Public Hygiene**

- Increase the number of health centres capable of dealing with surgical abdominal emergencies, in order to reduce delays in consultations.
- Move towards health pooling and universal health insurance, to facilitate access to healthcare for the population and reduce delays in consultations.

o **To the Director General of the Centre Hospitalier Universitaire Yalgado Ouédraogo**

- Make all operating theatres operational in order to prevent delays in treatment.
- Fitting out archive rooms to ensure that data is properly stored gross.

o **Medical staff**

- Ensure that medical documents are properly maintained.
- Fill in medical documents and keep them up to date.

o **To the public**

- Respect the highway code and the rules of social conduct.
- Consult the nearest health centre immediately after any trauma.

REFERENCES

1. **Abdallah A**. Abdomen: Wall and peritoneum. Cours polycopié destiné aux étudiants de la 2ème année médecine. faculté de médecine, département de médecine, La boratoire médico-chirurgicale; 2009 p4.

2. **André T, Arvieux C, Barbois S, Baratte C, Benchimol D, Benizri E, et al. General, visceral and digestive surgery. MED-LINE. Editions; 2022. 349 p. (Collège Français de Chirurgie Générale, Viscérale et Digestive Conseil National des Universités de Chirurgie Viscérale et Digestive).**

3. **Attiou EO**. Abdominal wounds caused by firearms at Tengandogo University Hospital: Epidemiological, clinical, paraclinical, therapeutic and evolutionary aspects. A propos de 38 cas. [Thèse de médecine]. [Ouagadougou]: Université Joseph Ki-Zerbo; 2020, 146p.

4. **Belemlilga GLH, Zaré C, Yabré N, Keita N, Benao BL, Somé OR, et al.** Abdominal Trauma in Africa: Epidemiological, Diagnostic, and Therapeutic Aspects. 2020;10. Available from: URL:http://dx.doi.org/10.19044/esj.2020.v16n21p132

5. **Benlaldj A**. Acute peritonitis. In: Enseignement de Chirurgie digestive à la faculté de médecine de Mostaganem. EPH de Mostaganem Algérie; 2016. p. 29.

6. **Bombah Freddy, Biwolé Daniel, Ekani Boukar, NgoNonga Bernadette, Essomba Arthur**. Prise en Charge Chirurgicales des Plaies Pénétrantes Abdominales à l'Hôpital Laquintinie de Douala: Indications, Techniques et Résultats à Propos de 37 Cas. 2020;21:7.

7. **Boubir SM**. Trauma of the abdomen. Module des urgences médico-chirurgicales 6 ème année Médecine. Universite Hadj Lakhdar Batna2 Faculte De Medecine; 2020, 8p.

8. **Boukhatmi L**. Anatomy of the peritoneum. General anatomy Faculty of médecine d'Oran; 2017, 7p.

9. **Bouzat P, Valdenaire G, Gauss T, Charbit J, Arvieux C, Balandraud P, et al.** Recommendations Formalisées D'experts " Prise En Charge Du Traumatisme Abdominal Grave De L'adulte : Les 48 Premières Heures " The Early Management Of Severe Abdominal Trauma. RFE commune SFAR - SFMU en association avec : AFC, AFU, SFRI and EVG. 2019;31.

10. **CDU-HGE**. Item 275 Acute Peritonitis. In: Abrégé d'Hépato-Gastro-Entérologie. 2nd edition. France: Editions Elsevier-Masson; 2012. p. 11 (chapter 29).

11. **CDU-HGE**. Item 352 - UE 11 - Acute peritonitis in children and adults. In: Collégiale des universitaires en hépato-gastro-entérologie. 4th edition. France; 2018. p. 427-34 (Les référentiels des Collèges).

12. **CDU-HGE**. Subject 57 Acute Peritonitis: Physiopathology, Diagnosis, Therapeutic Orientations. In: Cours de résidanat. Tunisia: Faculté de médecine de Sfax; 2019. p. 24.

13. **Choua O**, **Ali MM**, **Kaboro M**, **Moussa K**, **Anour M**. Etiological, clinical, and therapeutic aspects of acute generalized peritonitis in N'Djamena, Chad. Medecine et Sante Tropicales. 1 Jul 2017;27:270-3.

14. **Choua O, Moussa K, N'Djanone K, Ahmat M, Aboulghassim O, Sadie I, et al**. Posttraumatic perforations of hollow viscera at the national referral general hospital in N'Djamena, Chad. 2019;19:7.

15. **Clements TW, Tolonen M, Ball CG, Kirkpatrick AW**. Secondary Peritonitis and Intra-Abdominal Sepsis: An Increasingly Global Disease in Search of Better Systemic Therapies. Scand J Surg. June 2021;110(2):139-49.

16. **Daboué RMFC**. Les péritonites aiguës généralisées post-traumatiques au Centre Hospitalier Universitaire Yalgado Ouédraogo au Burkina Faso : aspects épidémiologiques, cliniques, thérapeutiques et évolutifs [Thèse de médecine]. [Ouagadougou]: Joseph Ki-Zerbo University; 2016, 150p.

17. **Debbache H**. Peritonitis. In: Enseignement de sémiologie digestive. Université de Constantine 3: Faculté de médecine; 2020. p. 5.

18. **Diakité L**. Aiguës Péritonites Généralisées Aspects Epidémiologiques et Thérapeutiques a l'hôpital Alfousseyni Daou de Kayes [Thèse de médecine]. [Bamako]: Université des Sciences, des Techniques et des Technologies de Bamako (USTTB); 2014, 103p.

19. **Diamoutene N**. Traumatismes de l'abdomen : aspect épidémio-clinique et thérapeutique dans le service de chirurgie A du centre hospitalier universitaire du Point-G [thesis]. [Bamako]: Université Des Sciences Des Techniques Et Des Technologies De Bamako Faculté De Médecine Et D'odontostomatologie; 2021, 113p.

20. **Diarra L**. Traumatic perforations of the digestive tract in the general surgery department of the Pr. Bocar Sidi Sall University Hospital of Kati [Medical thesis]. [Mali]: Université des Sciences des Techniques et des Technologies de Bamako; 2023, 116p.

21. **Drake RL**, **Mitchell AWM**, **Vogl W**. Gray's Anatomy for Students. Elsevier Masson; 2006. 1111 p.

22. **Elasbahani Y**. Trauma to the abdomen [Thesis in medicine]. [Marrakech]: Cadi Ayyad University; 2020, 147p.

23. **F. Sabbah, L. Ifrine, M. Ahallat, S. Benamar, A. Hrora, R. Mssrori, et al.** Digestive surgical pathology. 4th year medicine course. Université Mohammed V Souissi Faculté de Médecine et de Pharmacie de Rabat; 2013, 152p.

24. **Harrois A, Hamada S, Laplace C, Duranteau J**. Abdominal trauma. Département d'Anesthésie-Réanimation, Hôpital de Bicêtre, 78, avenue du Général Leclerc, 94275 Le Kremlin Bicêtre, France [Internet].2017;27. Available from: https:Harrois-Traumatisme-abdominal.pdf

25. **Ilboudo F**. Peritonitis secondary to firm trauma of the abdomen: epidemiological, clinical, paraclinical, therapeutic and evolutionary aspects in the general and digestive surgery department of the Yalgado Ouédraogo University Hospital of Ouagadougou, Burkina Faso [Thèse de médecine]. [Ouagadougou]: Joseph Ki-Zerbo; 2019, 133p.

26. **Jean-Philippe D**. Atlas of general and radiological anatomy. 2nd edition. France: rue Camille-Desmoulins, 92442 Issy-les-Moulineaux cedex; 2019. 304 p. (Elsevier Masson SAS).

27. **Kaboré E**. Péritonites aiguës généralisées au Centre Hospitalier Universitaire Tengandogo : Aspects épidémiologiques, étiologiques, thérapeutiques, et pronostiques (à propos de 94 cas) [Thèse de médecine]. [Ouagadougou]: Université Joseph Ki-Zerbo; 2018, 135p.

28. **Kambiré JL, Ouédraogo S, Zida M, Ouédraogo S, Sanon BG**. Les traumatismes abdominaux : aspects épidémiologiques et lésionnels au centre hospitalier universitaire régional de Ouahigouya, Burkina Faso / abdominal trauma: epidemiological and lesional aspects at the regional teaching hospital center of Ouahigouya, Burkina Faso. 2018;5.

29. **Kamina P**. Clinical anatomy. Maloine. Vol. Tome3. 27, rue de l'école de médecine, 75006 Paris; 2009. 180 p.

30. **Kangudia M. J.** Special embryology course G3 BM | PDF | Pancreas | Peritoneum[Internet]. 2014 [cited 28 Jan 2023]. Available at: https://fr.scribd.com/document/619263505/Cours-d-embryologie-speciale- G3-BM

31. **Lasocki S, Gaillard T, Lemaire P, Leger M**. Peritonitis: the first hours! SFAR-Le Congrès.2018;20p.

32. **Magagi I. A., Adamou H., Habou O., Magagi A., Halidou M., Ganiou K. Emergencies surgical digestive in Africa: study prospective study of a series of 622 patients at Zinder National Hospital, Niger. Bull Soc Pathol Exot. March 2016;7.**

33. **Maiga B**. Péritonite Post Traumatique En Chirurgie Pédiatrique Au Chu Gabriel Toure [Thesis]. [Mali]: Université des Sciences, des Techniques et des Technologies de Bamako; 2022, 121p.

34. **Mouzou T, Egbonhou P, Tomta K, Bissang AK**. Abdominal trauma at the Sylvanus Olympio University Hospital in Lomé. - Société de l'Anesthésie Réanimation d'Afrique Francophone. July 2014; https://web-saraf.net/?Traumatismes-abdominaux-au-CHU.

35. **Ouahab I**. Péritonites aiguës. cours. Université Ferhat Abbas De Setif Faculté De Médecine; 2020, 18p.

36. **Ouangré E, Zida M, Bonkoungou GP, Sanou A, Traore S**. Les Péritonites Aigües Généralisées en milieu rural au Burkina Faso: A propos de 221 cas. dec 2013;1(2):5.

37. **Ouattara S**. Support de cours Doctorat 1 de médecine: Organisation des services de santé. UJKZ; 2021, 115p.

38. **Ouédraogo B**. Cinquième Recensement Général de la Population et de l'Habitation du Burkina Faso [Internet]. Institut National de la Statistique et de la Démographie; 2022. Available at: www.insd.bf

39. **Ouédraogo I**. Traumatic wounds of the abdomen: epidemiological, aetiological, lesional, therapeutic and evolutionary aspects in two health structures in the city of Ouagadougou. [Thèse de médecine]. [Ouagadougou]: Joseph Ki-Zerbo; 2020, 138p.

40. **Pérrigault F, Gauzit R**. Intra-abdominal infection: how to treat in 2015. Paris Descartes University. 10 June 2015;87.

41. **Philippe Montravers, Hervé Dupont, Marc Leone, Jean-Michel Constantin, Paul-Michel Mertes**. Management of intraabdominal infections. Société française d'anesthésie et de réanimation. feb 2015;tom1:75-99.

42. **Philippe Montravers, Sylvain Jean-Baptiste, Parvine Tashk**. Peritonitis. Department of Anaesthesia and Intensive Care, CHU Bichat Claude-Bernard - HUPNVS. 2016;20.

43. **Raherinantenaina F, Rakotomena SD, Rajaonarivony T, Rabetsiahiny LF, Rajaonanahary TMA, Rakototiana FA, et al.** Closed and penetrating trauma of the abdomen: retrospective analysis on 175 cases and review of the literature. feb 2015;10.

44. **Richard L Drake, A Wayne Vogl, Adam W M Mitchell**. Gray's anatomy. the textbook for students. 4th edition. France: rue Camille-Desmoulins, 92442 Issy-les-Moulineaux cedex; 2020. 1178 p. (Elsevier Masson; vol. 1178).

45. **Sambo BT, Hodonou AM, Allode AS, Mensah E, Youssouf M, Menhinto D. Epidemiological, Diagnostic And Therapeutic Aspects Of Abdominal Trauma In Bembéréké-North Benin. European Scientific Journal March**

2016 edition. 2016;12(9):11.

46. **Sergiy K**. Epidemiology and Management of Peritonitis at a Rural Hospital in Zambia. Sept 2020;17(3):120-5.

47. **Si A**. Anatomy of the peritoneum for medical courses. Department D'anatomie Normale CHU Oran; 2015, 34p.

48. **Sogoba G, Katilé D, Sangaré S, Traoré L, Diakité L, Cissé S, et al.** Clinical Presentation, Treatment and Evolution of Acute Generalized Peritonitis at the Fousseyni Daou Hospital in Kayes, Mali. June 2021;22(6):58-61.

49. **Sylla D**. Perforations Digestives Traumatiques Dans Le Service De Chirurgie Générale De L'hôpital De Sikasso [Thesis in medicine]. [Mali]: Université des Sciences, des Techniques et des Technologies de Bamako; 2021, 113p.

50. **Thiam A**. Centre du Mali: Enjeu et danger d'une crise négligée. Mali: Institut du Macina; 2017 March p. 60.

51. **Tochie JN, Agbor NV, Frank Leonel TT, Mbonda A, Abang DA, Danwang C**. Global epidemiology of acute generalised peritonitis: a protocol for a systematic review and meta-analysis. BMJ Open 2020;10:e034326. Jan 2020;4.

52. **Ulrych J, Zeman M, Adamkova V**. Post-traumatic peritonitis [Internet]. [cited 15 Jan 2023]. Available from: https:post-traumatic-peritonitis-109333

53. **Yabi OG**. General presentation of Burkina Faso. Fiche pays [Internet]. Wathinotes. 6 Nov 2020 [quoted 20 Oct 2022]; Available from at: https://www.wathi.org/contexte-election-burkina-2020/presentation- generale-du-burkina-faso/

54. **Yao O**. Ranking of African countries according to their HDI in 2021 [Internet]. sikafinance.com. [cited 20 Oct 2022]. Available from: https://www.sikafinance.com/marches/classement-des-pays-africains-selon- leur-idh-en-2021_36587

Collection form

Post-traumatic peritonitis in the general and digestive surgery department of the CHU-YO from 05 april 2019 to 04 april 2022

Collection form N°

A. General information

Patient identity

File N°/ / **Initials** / /**Age** / / **Sex** / / **Residence :**Rural/ /Urban/ / **Occupation:** Informal sector / / Employed / / Pupil/student / / Farmer/breeder / / FAF / / Other (please specify) //

Admission to emergency surgery

Date and time of entry / / / / à /H /min **Mode of admission:** Direct / / Referral / / Transfer / / **Referral structure:** CHU/ / CHR / / CMA / / FS privée //

B. Clinical data

Reason for consultation or reference

Wound penetrating//**Evisceration**//**Contusion**/   /

Other / / Indeterminate / **Indeterminate** //

History of the disease

Date of injury / / / / **Time /min Consultation time: <6h** / / 6h - 12h / />12h/   /

Mechanism of occurred MVA / RTA / / Type : Auto - Auto / / Auto –   Moto / / Moto - Moto / / Moto - Obstacle / / Auto –   Obstacle / / **Assault** / / Type : Firearm / / White weapon / / Other / /

Sports accident / / Foot ball / / Other / / **Work accident** / / Type / / Other / / Specify / / Sports **accident** / **Other** / / Specify //History

Medical: Yes / / No / / Specify / / **Surgical:** Yes / / No / / Specify /

/ **Mode et habitude de vie :** Alcool / / Tabac / / Café / /

General signs

General condition WHO stage: II / / **III** / / I V /**State of consciousness:** Normal / / Dazed / / Comatose / / **Colour of conjunctiva:** Normal / / Pale / / Icteric / / **Fold of malnutrition:** Yes /_ / No /_ / **Fold of dehydration:** Yes /_/ No /_ / **Vitals:** Temperature: Lowered / / Normal/ / Elevated / / Blood pressure: Lowered / / Normal/ / Elevated / / Heart rate: Lowered / / Normal/ / Elevated / / Respiratory rate: Lowered / / Normal/ / Elevated / / **Shock:** Yes / / No / / / No

Physical signs

Inspection

Abdominal distension: Yes /_/ No /_/ Ecchymosis: Yes /_/ No /_/ Abdominal wound: Yes /_/ No /_/ Site of injury /./ **Palpation**

Contractureabdominale :Yes/_/No/_/ Abdominal defence:Localized/_/Generalized/_/ Umbilical cry: Yes /_/ No /_/ Abdominal mass: Yes /_/ No /_ **Percussion**

Normal // Dullness // Tympany / /

Auscultation

Normal // Abdominal silence / /

Touchrectal

Normal / / Douglas fir cry //

Polytrauma / /Other injuries

C.Paraclinical signs Biology

Leucocytes: Lowered//Normal//High // **Haemoglobin level:** Low//Normal/ /
Blood glucose: Lowered//Normal// High// **Creatinemia:** Normal / / High / /
Blood urea: Normal / / High / / **Ion disorder:** Yes /_/No /_/ Specify: / /
Imaging
ASP: Yes /_/ No /_/ Result: Normal /_/ Hydroaerobic level /_/ Gas crescent / / Diffuse greyness / /

Ultrasound : Yes /_/ No /_/ Result : Normal // Haemoperitoneum / / **CT scan:** Yes /_/ No /_/ Result: Normal / / Gas crescent / / Fluid effusion / /

D.Intraoperative diagnosis: Post-traumatic peritonitis
Abdominal contusion /_/ Penetrating wound /_/ Traumatic evisceration /_/ Ballistic wound /_/ Other // Indeterminate /_/

E. Treatment Medical treatment
Preoperative resuscitation: Yes /_/ No /_/ Venous catheter / / Urinary catheter / / Nasogastric catheter / / Oxygen / / Intubation catheter / / Blood transfusion /_/ Quantity Vascular filling /_/ Quantity: Rehydration / /Quantity:
Analgesics: Nefopam / / Paracetamol / / Tramadol / / Morphine /_/ **Antibiotics:** Injectable / / Ceftriaxone / / Metronidazole / / Ampicillin / / Gentamycune /_/ Amoxicillin clavulanic acid /_/ **Tetanus serotherapy /_/.**
Post-operative resuscitation: Blood transfusion // Quantity :
Vascular filling /_/ Quantity : Rehydration /_/ Quantity:**Analgesics:** Nefopa/ / Paracetamol // Tramadol/ Morphine // **Antibiotic:** Injectable / / Ceftriaxone /   /

Metronidazole // Ampicillin
/ Gentamycune / / Amoxicillin clavulanic acid / / Oral /_/ Ciprofloxacin /_ /
Amoxicillin /_ / Metronidazole /_ / **Anticoagulant /_ / Anti-inflammatory /_ /
PPI** / /

Treatmentsurgical

Date and time o f operation / / / at / H min **Time taken for surgical
management: <24h / / 24h - 48h /_ / >48h / / Duration of operation / / Type
of anaesthesia:** GA / / ALR / / **Type of operation:** Laparotomy / / Laparoscopy
/ / **Approach:** Midline / / Other // **State of abdominal cavity:** Clean / /
Serohematic fluid / / Serous fluid / / Citrin fluid / / Pus / / Fecaloid / / Bilious / /
Other (specify) () Quantité / /

Damaged organs: Stomach / / Duodenum / / Jejunum / / Ileum / / Colon / /
Rectum / / Gall bladder / / Liver / / Spleen / / Pancreas / / Bladder / / Liver / /
Spleen / / Pancreas / / Bladder / / Kidney / / Kidney / / Kidney / / Kidney / /
Kidney / Kidney / Kidney / Kidney / Kidney / Kidney /Kidney//Other(specify)//()

Type of injury / /

Procedures performed: Suture // Excision suture / / Ileostomy // Colostomy/ /
Jejunal resection / / Ileal resection / / Colonic resection / / Anastomosis
//Splenectomy/ / Removal fossae membrane//Toilet peritoneal// Other / /
Associated procedure (specify) // () **Intraoperative incident and accident**
(specify) / / () **Evolution**

Post-op : Simple//Complicated// **General complications:** Sepsis / / Pressure
sores / / Haemorrhage / / Other // **Specific complications:** parietal suppuration //
Evisceration / / Post-operative peritonitis / / Digestive fistula / Digestive fistula/
/ Stomal prolapse // Post-operative occlusion / / Phagedema   / Phagedenism / /
Other // **Resumption in the operating theatre:** Yes /_ / No /_ / Number of
times: 1 /_ / 2 /_ / >2 /_ /

F. Output

Date and time of output ////à/HMin **Durée d'hospitalisation : <5j /_ / 5 – 10j
/_ / 10 – 20j /_ / >20j /_ / Modalité de sortie :** Guéri / / Lost to follow-up / /
Referred / /Died/ /**Siderectomy:**Peroperative// Postoperative/Probable cause of
death / **Follow-up consultation** / /

ICONOGRAPHY

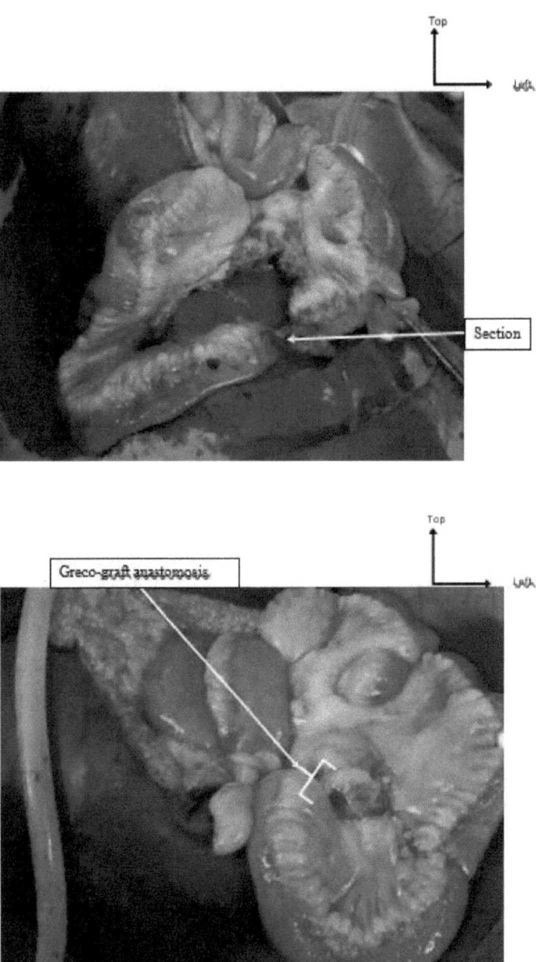

Figure 9: Section of the small intestine and its mesentery following closed abdominal trauma after a road traffic accident in a young patient (Image from the general and digestive surgery department of the CHU-YO 2021).

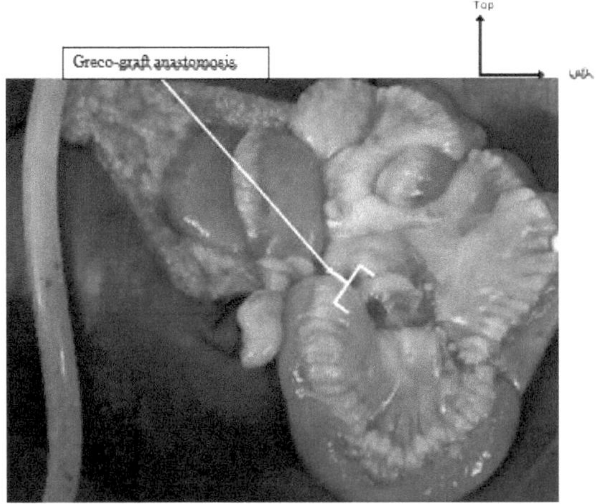

Figure 10: Greco-grenic anastomosis (Image of the general and digestive surgery department at CHU-YO 2021)

HIPPOCRATIC OATH

In the presence of the masters of this school and my fellow students, I promise and swear to befaithful to the laws of honour and probity in the practice of medicine. I will give my care free of charge to the needy and I will never demand a salary above my work. When admitted to the interior of houses, my eyes will not see what goes on there; my tongue will keep silent about the secrets entrusted to me and my status will not be used to corrupt morals or encourage crime. Respectful and grateful to my masters, I will give their children the instruction I received from their fathers. May men esteem me if I have remained faithful to my promises, and may I be covered with opprobrium

SUMMARY

Title: *Post-traumatic peritonitis in the General and Digestive Surgery Department of the CHU-YO in Burkina Faso*

Objective : *Studying post-traumatic peritonitis in the general and digestive surgery department of the CHU-YO from April 01, 2019 to March 31, 2022*

Method and patients : *This was a descriptive retrospective study over a period of three years, from April 01, 2019 to March 31, 2022.*

Results: *Peritonitis occurred in 34.14% of abdominal trauma and accounted for 08.02% of acute generalized peritonitis. 50% of these peritonitis occurred from August to November. The mean age of the patients was 30.39 years with a sex ratio of 17.66. The informal sector represented 42.85% and the reference was the most frequent mode of admission 75%, from the CMA. Traffic accidents accounted for 44.64% followed by assaults, 41.07%. Abdominal contracture was only found in 17.85% of cases. The rarely requested ASP x-ray found 100% of a gaseous crescent. The small intestine was the injured organ in 82.14% of cases, of which the jejunum represented 58.82%. The surgical gesture was therefore a suture resection of the small intestine in 39.28% of cases and an anastomotic resection in 37.50%.*

Conclusion : *Post traumatic peritonitis is relatively common. It is dominated by road accidents. The small intestine is the most damaged organ. Maintenance of the road network and sensitization of the population on compliance with the highway code could contribute to reducing this scourge.*

***Key words** : Peritonitis - Road accident - Jejunum - CHU-YO*

Author: *Ira Issouf iraissuf@gmail.comPhone: (+226) 64568103*